Published by Reflections Publishing
© 2012 Reflections Publishing.

First Edition. Published in the United States of America.

ISBN 978-1-61660-012-9

Visit our web site at www.reflectionspublishing.com for more information or inquiries.

* * *

Other books by Reflections Publishing:

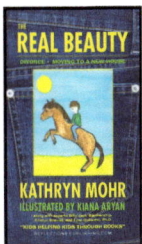

The Real Beauty: Navigating Through Divorce and Moving
ISBN: 978-1-61660-000-6
Written by: Kathryn Mohr
Illustrated by: Kiana Aryan

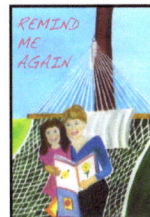

Remind Me Again: Navigating Through the Loss of a Loved One
HC: ISBN: 978-1-61660-001-3
P: ISBN: 978-1-61660-010-5
Written by: The Ster Family
Illustrated by: Colleen C. Ster

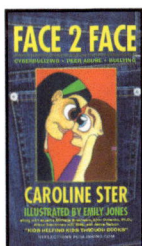

Face 2 Face: Navigating Through Cyberbullying, Peer Abuse, & Bullying
ISBN: 978-1-61660-002-0
Written by: Caroline Ster
Illustrated by: Emily Jones

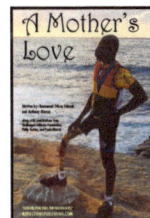

A Mother's Love: Overcoming a Disability and Believing in Yourself
HC: ISBN: 978-1-61660-011-2
P: ISBN: 978-1-61660-008-2
Written by: Anthony Mazza & Emmanuel Ofosu Yeboah

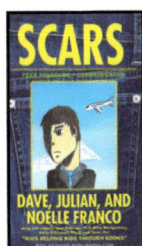

Scars: Navigating Through Peer Pressure & Consequences of Actions
ISBN: 978-1-61660-003-7
By Parent/Child Team:
Dave, Julian, and Noelle Franco

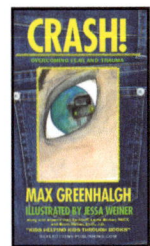

Crash: Overcoming Fear and Trauma
ISBN: 978-1-61660-006-8
Written by: Max Greenhalgh
Illustrated by: Jessa Weiner

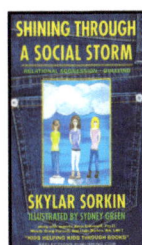

Shining Through a Social Storm: Navigating Through Relational Aggression, Bullying, and Popularity
ISBN: 978-1-61660-004-4
Written by: Skylar Sorkin
Illustrated by: Sydney Green

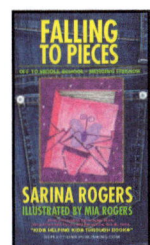

Falling to Pieces: Navigating the Transition to Middle School and Merging Friends
ISBN: 978-1-61660-007-5
Written by: Sarina Rogers
Illustrated by: Mia Rogers

Dedications:

I dedicate this book to my supporting family. To my older sister, Caroline, my twin sister, Alexandra, my mom and dad, my Papa Jerry, and my dog Angel.
—Isabelle Angelite Ster

I dedicate this book to my grandfather, Bill Bohan, who loves me unconditionally.
—Emily Morgan

To all my patients living with dementia and their families.
—John W. Daly, M.D.

I dedicate this book to all the students I've had during my teaching career. You have all taught me precious life lessons along the way.
—Jennifer McClellan

For my grandmother, Margaret Anderson, who with Alzheimer's Disease, did not remember many things, but always remembered her Lord and His love for her! What a comfort!
—Cindy Wright

To my dad, Jerry, thank you for letting me walk alongside you during this journey.
—Colleen Carter Ster

Charity:

A portion of sales from this book will be donated to the Alzheimer's Association (alz.org).

Sales:

The student author and illustrator of this book will be distributing a portion of their earnings into their college savings funds.

Remember Me When

Isabelle Angelite Ster
Illustrated by Emily Morgan

along with Dr. John Daly,
Jennifer McClellan, M.A.,
and Cindy Wright

Remember me even when I don't remember you.

Talk to me about things from long ago because my last memories are from years ago.

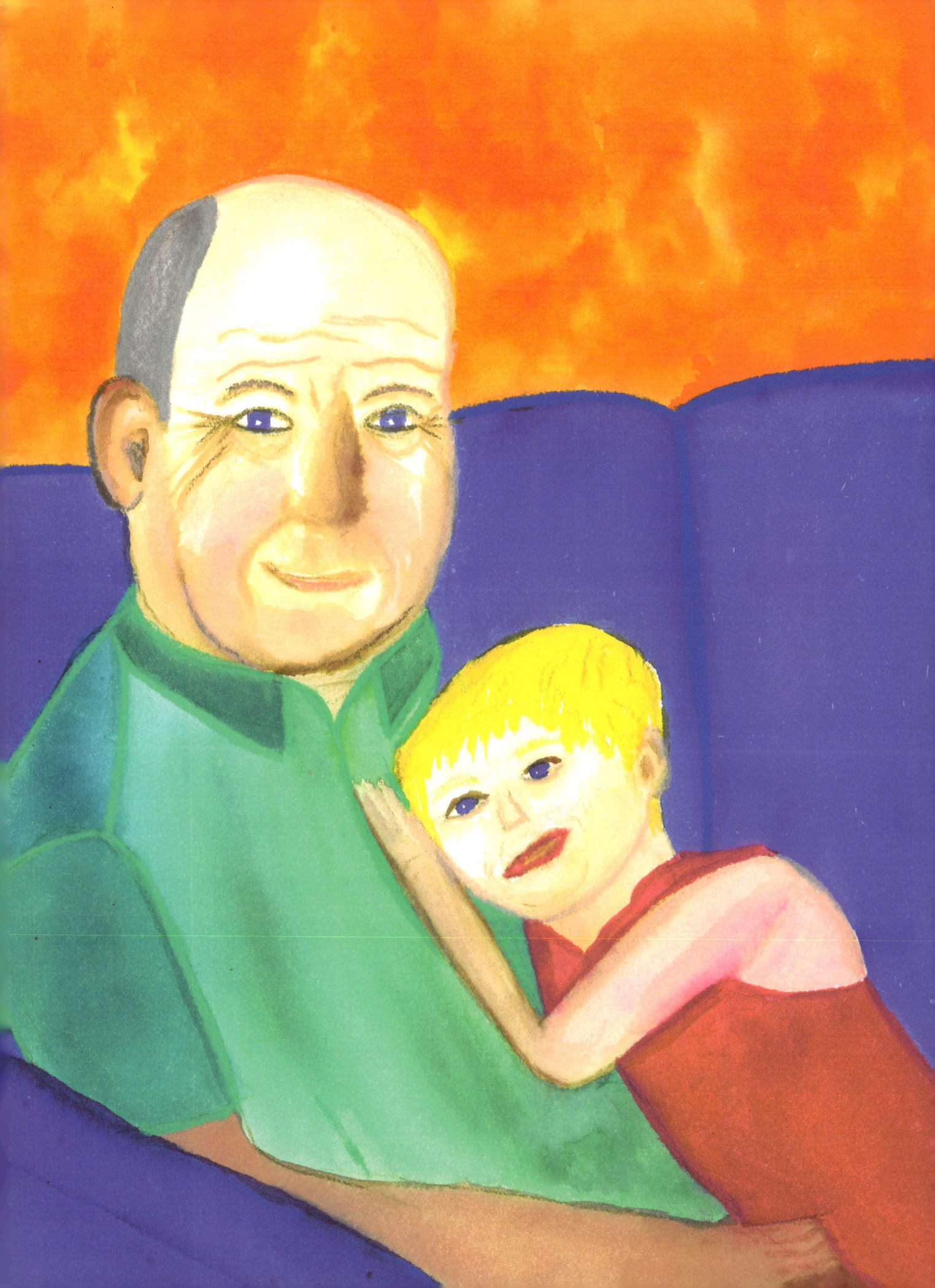

Sometimes my thoughts are not always clear. I may tell people you play guitar when you actually play violin, or I may claim to know famous people I have never even met.

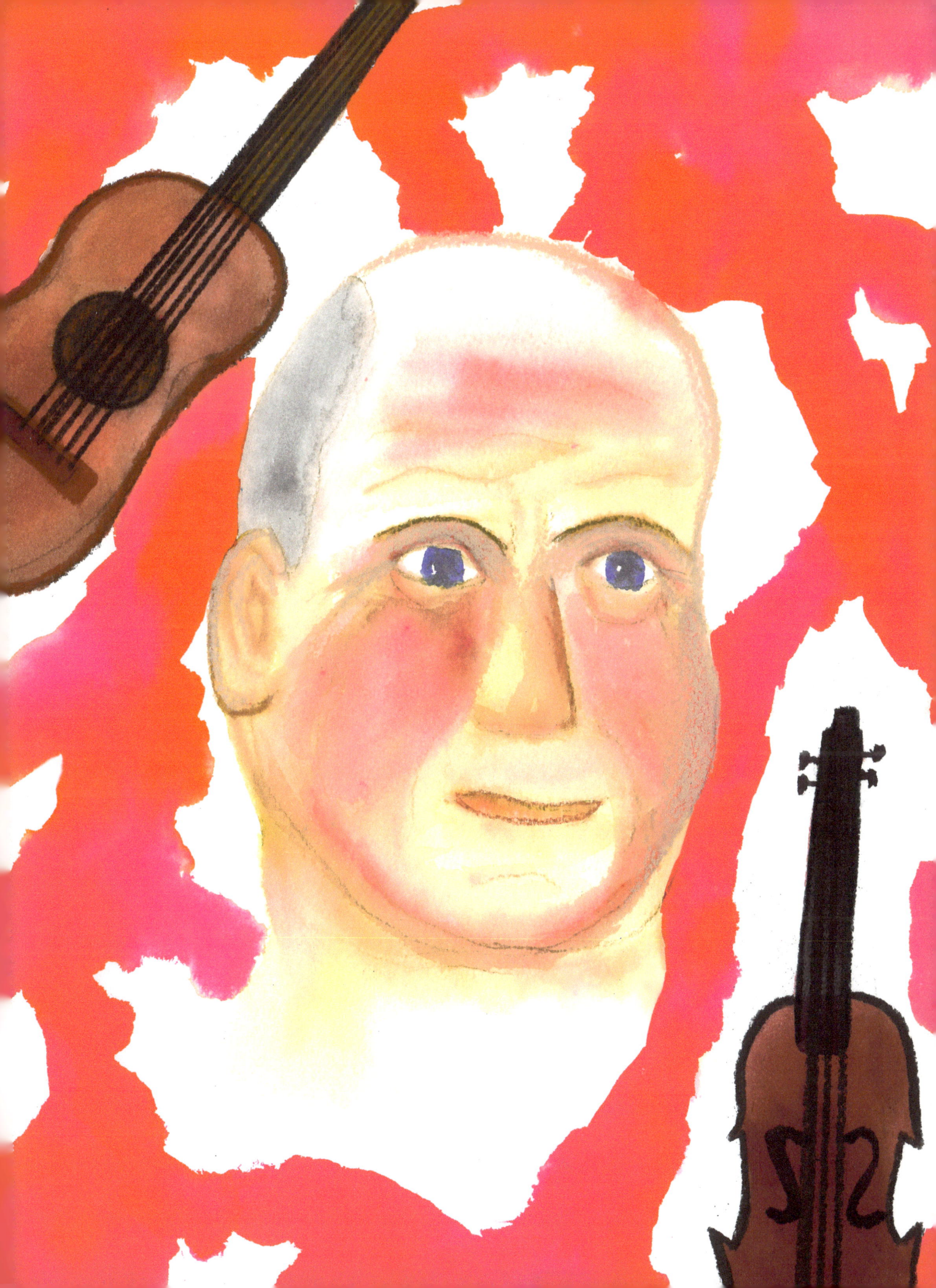

As my brain unwinds, it unwinds like a ball of yarn, so any new information is the first to go.

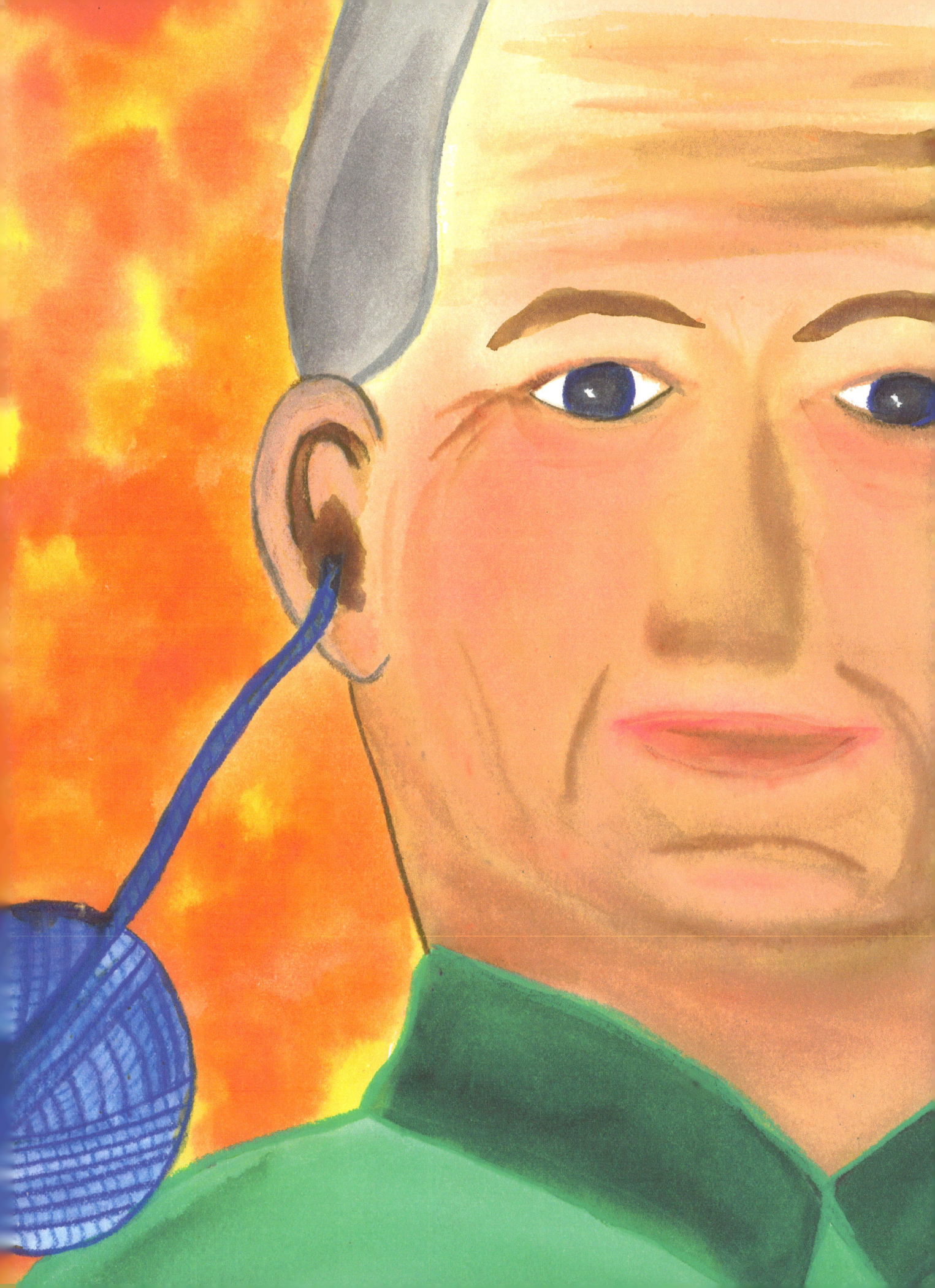

I don't love you less because I don't remember you. Now, I just remember you as the person dressed in bright clothes or jewels that sparkle, or as the person with the big smile, or as someone who will give me a big bear hug.

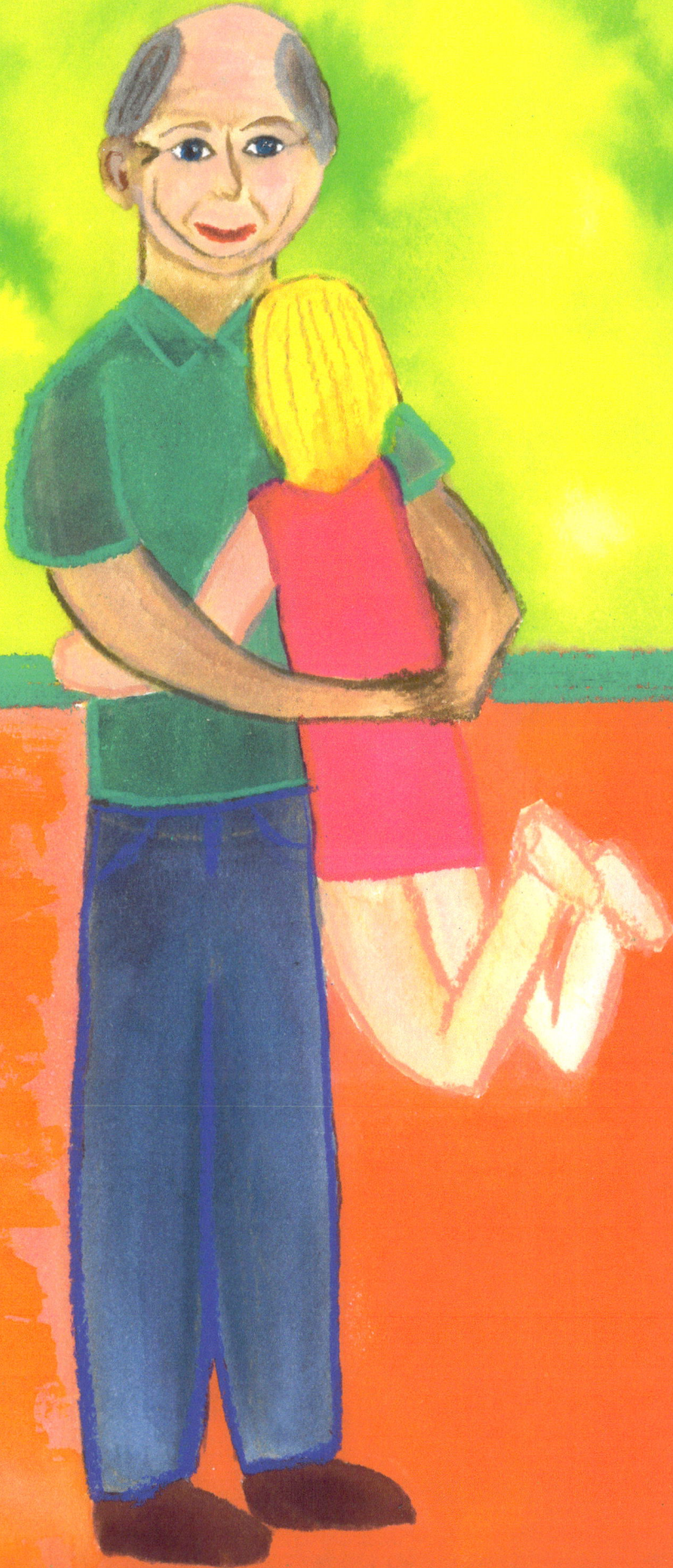

Don't be sad for me. You don't want me to suffer. Be happy for me when I move on to a better place and God makes me whole again.

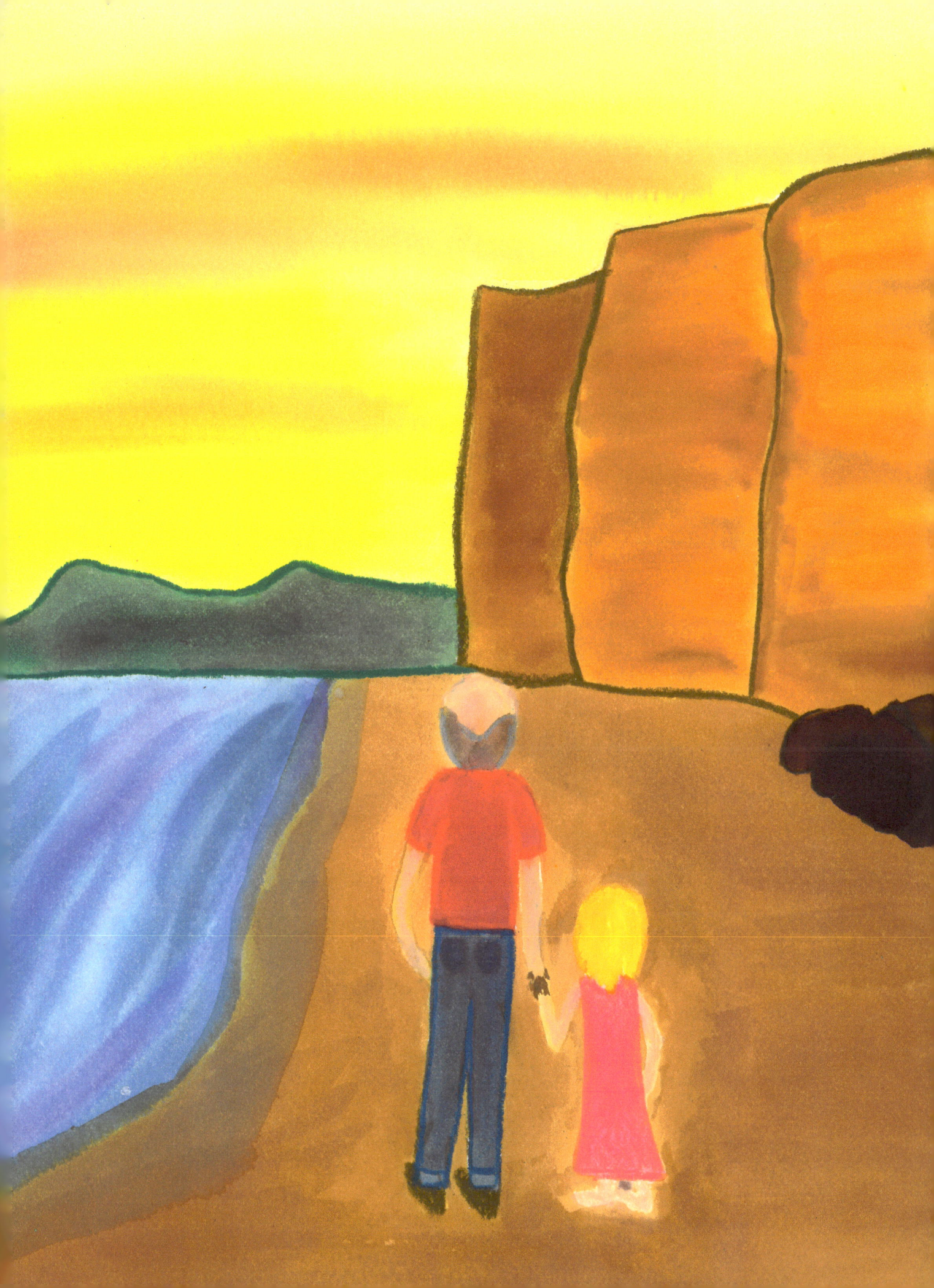

Even though, someday, I may not remember you—I will always love you day-to-day, week-to-week, and year-to-year.

You will always be in my heart.

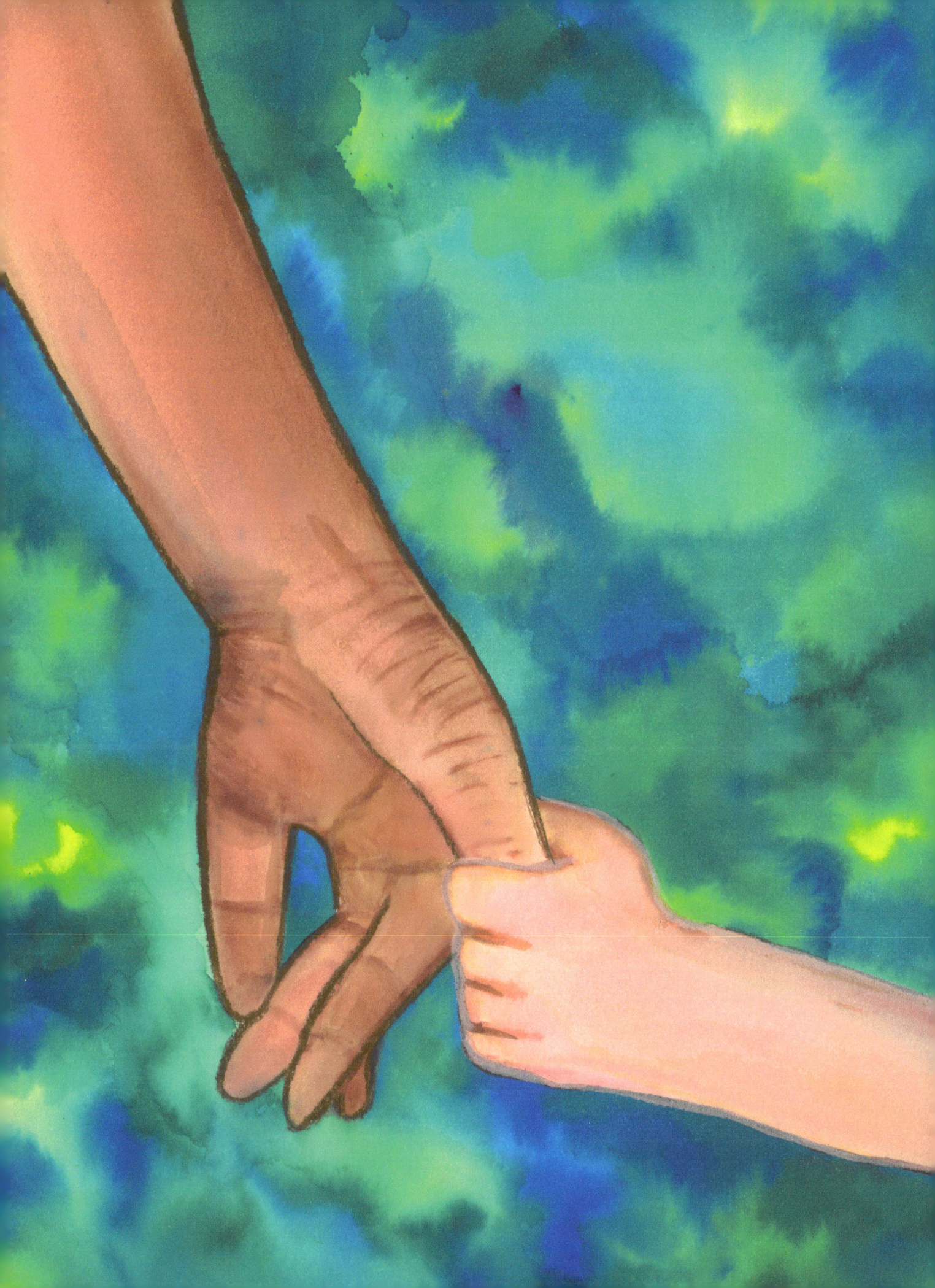

4114U
(Information For You!)

Each book in Reflections Publishing's "Kids Helping Kids Through Books" series comes with a support system of how to help families to heal emotionally, socially, and spiritually through each difficult life challenge. *Remember Me When*, written by Isabelle Ster, is a heartfelt story that was created as she was navigating ways to communicate with her Papa Jerry as he progressed through Alzheimer's disease.

Alzheimer's disease is a difficult journey, but listed below are some positive ways to interact with your loved one.

10 Helpful Interactive Tips

1. Take family photos to display around your loved one's room.

2. Give your loved one a big bear hug each time you see them.

3. Wear bright-colored clothing or an item that shimmers and sparkles to stimulate their sense of sight.

4. Bring picture books of activities they have always enjoyed such as bird watching or gardening, and tape a picture of yourself in the front of the book with your name written below to help stimulate their memory.

5. Schedule regular appointments to get their hair cut, or to receive a manicure, pedicure, or massage.

6. Bring a game or activity such as flower arranging to do with your loved one.

7. Always wear a smile because they will sense how you are feeling. Share your joy and laughter with them.

8. Take them out to dinner or join them for a meal and make sure you get dessert. Your loved one likely has a sweet tooth now.

9. Talk to them about their childhood and early memories because they will remember those times the best.

10. Tell them that you love them and gently rub their back. This is very soothing and calming for both of you. If they become anxious, have a phrase ready to confidently say such as, "Everything is going to be okay. We are all in this together."

Action Steps to Help Families Emotionally

Written by:
John W. Daly, M.D.
Clinical Professor, Geriatric Medicine, UCSD
Program Director, UCSD Geriatric Medicine Fellowship Program

What is Alzheimer's disease?

Alzheimer's disease is a disease of the brain. It is one of the brain diseases called dementia. Dementia affects how we remember, think, and behave. As the disease progresses, a material called amyloid forms plaques in the brain, and this causes normal brain cells (called neurons) to deteriorate and become tangles of a material called tau. When this happens, these areas of the brain no longer function normally.

The part of the brain first involved with Alzheimer's disease controls how we remember things, and the loss of memory is one of the first signs of the illness. As the disease progresses, other areas of the brain are affected, and the person may lose the ability to solve problems, recognize family members, or take care of one's self.

Because the disease gets worse over time, it is often described as having a progression through 3 different stages: mild, moderate, and severe.

The Stages of Alzheimer's disease

MILD
- Repeating questions
- Forgetting plans for the day
- Losing things

MODERATE
- Problems with usual tasks
- Difficulty paying bills and shopping
- Problems driving

SEVERE
- Problems dressing self
- Problems feeding self
- Difficulty walking

In the mild stage, the person with Alzheimer's disease has problems with short-term memory. This means they forget things that may have just happened. In this stage, the person and their family may not even know that the disease is starting. In the mild stage, the person may also repeat the same question over and over because they forget it has been asked. They may forget the plans that have been made for the day or get lost in a familiar place. In this stage, the person might misplace or lose things and think that their items have been stolen. They also may become easily frustrated or angry at times.

In the moderate stage, it is common for one to have problems with usual daily tasks. The person with Alzheimer's disease may forget to pay their bills and have problems with shopping. They may have difficulty with cooking or doing other things that they used to be able to do well. Driving becomes more difficult, and one may become lost or have car accidents. They might even mix up the names of their children or grandchildren, and forget important things like birthdays or holidays. The person with the illness is often not aware that they have problems and will think they are doing things in a normal way. They may respond to you differently and be more irritable. It is important to remember it is the disease doing this and not anything you have done to cause their anger. This is a difficult time for family members of the person with Alzheimer's disease.

In the severe stage, one loses the ability to perform basic care activities such as getting dressed, feeding one's self or taking a bath without assistance. At this stage of the disease, it can also become difficult for the person to walk safely without help, and there is a greater risk for falling and getting injured. At this point in the progression of the disease, the person requires care 24 hours a day, and often families need additional help with providing care.

Ways to help a family member with early (mild) stage Alzheimer's disease (AD):

There are several things you can do to help ease the frustration of someone who has early stage Alzheimer's disease. The most important thing is to remember that repeated questions or difficulties with tasks are part of the illness and not the fault of the person with the illness. Usually they are not aware of the changes they are experiencing. It is important to be patient and supportive, and not contribute to the frustration your loved one is experiencing. Do not become annoyed by repeated questions, but simply respond and move on to another topic.

A few basic suggestions to follow are:

1. Focus on one's successes, not their failures. Help your family member with AD engage in those tasks they can do well, and assist when they have difficulty. It is better to assist with something than to take it over completely.
2. Do not test them by asking questions about things they are having difficulty remembering, as this can increase frustration. A good example is to not keep asking what the date is if this is something they have a hard time remembering.
3. Remember that a touch and a smile often say much more than words.
4. It is difficult for the person with AD to start activities at times, and help is often needed and usually welcome.
5. Simple tasks may take a longer time to get done. Don't rush!
6. Talk with your parents, brothers, sisters, and friends about anything that makes you uncomfortable or scares you. It is normal to experience these feelings, and sharing them with loved ones can help.

For evaluation of patients, a good starting place is with the U.S. Department of Health and Human Services: Alzheimer's Disease Research Centers. Call 1-800-438-4380 or email: adear@nia.nih.gov

Action Steps to Help Families Socially

Written by:
Jennifer McClellan, M.A.
Second-Grade Teacher, Del Mar Union Schools

There is no doubt that dealing with any loss is challenging for a family. Alzheimer's disease is a double whammy, since you lose the person before they are gone. It can be a difficult concept for your child to understand that Grandpa or Grandma is here, but his/her mind works differently now. When kids are confused, it can upset him/her in their daily life. It is extremely important that you open up to your child's teacher if something like this is happening to your family. Many times, their school day is the only thing that stays consistent, which creates a safe feeling when things at home have been turned upside down.

"Teacher, Teacher!"

"411" for Children: Ways to Involve Your Teacher

1. Be a tattletale: Tell your teacher (and other appropriate adults) about the situation at home. This allows your teacher to understand why you might be more frustrated, sad, withdrawn, or having trouble concentrating at school.

2. Journal: Ask your teacher if you can spend time journaling your feelings if you are having a tough day. Expressing your feelings through words can help you to process how you are grieving the change your family is experiencing.

3. Go to the library: Ask your teacher if you can go to the library to find books on Alzheimer's disease. Often, we feel better when we research a topic and feel like we are better informed.

"411" for Parents: Ways to Involve the Teacher

1. Open up: Tell your teacher (and other appropriate adults) about the situation at home. This allows your teacher to monitor and connect with your child on a daily basis.

2. Checking in: Ask for periodic updates from the teacher on your child's ability to cope.

3. Family Bumps: Keep the teacher updated and alert to changes within the family dynamic. Many times, teachers have been through a similar situation and can relate to what your family is going through.

MOST OF ALL, stay in touch with your own feelings so you can clearly express them to the teacher. The knowledge you give the teacher will assist them in being a supporting team member for you and your family as you journey through this disease.

Action Steps to Help Families Spiritually

Written by:
Cindy Wright, Director of Mature Adults
Solana Beach Presbyterian Church

Your house of worship may be a valuable resource in finding support for your loved one with Alzheimer's disease or other forms of dementia. Consider the programs and services offered through your "senior ministries" program. Many senior ministries are geared for all levels of cognition and activity. Many places of worship offer support groups for caregivers, grief groups, and may host outside support groups as well. You may find that one's house of worship is a place of comfort and familiarity.

Keeping your loved one involved as he or she faces the challenges of their illness can be a source of encouragement. You don't need to reinvent the wheel in finding positive, effective ways to assist you in caring for your loved one. Places to go:

1. Your county will offer resources for older adults and have a variety of programs available. The Alzheimer's Association has regional offices with a multitude of family support options, classes, respite care, and helpful hints.

2. Many local police or sheriff's departments are equipped to provide safety and wellness checks as well as "safe return" programs in case your loved one should wander. The local senior center will have resources specific to your area that can be invaluable. Give them a call.

Lastly, remember with Alzheimer's' disease, your loved one may not remember what was eaten for lunch, but will be more familiar with early memories. Venture back to his or her youth with songs from Sunday School, old familiar hymns, and favorite scripture verses they have heard since childhood to recall the truths of God's everlasting love. Although one day your loved one may not know his or her name (or yours), our faithful God always loves and never forgets His children.

Here are a couple of favorite verses to help reassure your loved one of God's unfailing love:

- **Psalm 100:5** For the LORD is good and his love endures forever; his faithfulness continues through all generations.

- **Psalm 9:10** Those who know your name trust in you, for you, LORD, have never forsaken those who seek you.

References:

References for Adults:

- Coste, Joanne Koenig. *Learning to Speak Alzheimer's: A Groundbreaking Approach for Everyone Dealing with the Disease.* New York: Mariner Books, 2004.

- Genova, Lisa. *Still Alice.* New York: Pocket Books, 2009.

- Peterson, Barry. *Jan's Story.* California: Behler Publications, 2010.

- Shenk, David. *The Forgetting: Alzheimer's Portrait of an Epidemic.* New York: Knopf Doubleday Publishing Group, 2003.

References for Children (Grade Level):

- Schnurbush, Barbara. *Striped Shirts and Flowered Pants: A Story about Alzheimer's Disease for Young Children.* Washington, D.C.: Magination Press, 2007. **(all ages)**

- Shriver, Maria. *What's Happening to Grandpa?* New York: Little Brown, 2004. **(all ages)**

- Stickels, Terry. *Alzheimer's Association: The Big Brain Puzzle Book.* New York: Time Home Entertainment, 2009. **(all ages)**

Web Links:

- Alzheimer's Association
  www.alz.org

- KidsHealth from Nemours
  http://kidshealth.org/kid/grownup/conditions/alzheimers.html

- Mayo Clinic
  http://www.mayoclinic.com/health/alzheimers/HQ00216

- U.S. Department of Health and Human Services: Alzheimer's Disease Research Centers
  http://www.nia.nih.gov/alzheimers/alzheimers-disease-research-centers

Reflection Journal

Reflection Journal

Reflection Journal

www.ingramcontent.com/pod-product-compliance
Lightning Source LLC
Chambersburg PA
CBHW042002100426
42813CB00019B/2957